37444000125839

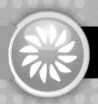

21st Century Skills **INNOVATION** *Library*

Hearing

by Susan H. Gray

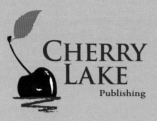

CHERRY
LAKE
Publishing

Published in the United States of America by Cherry Lake Publishing
Ann Arbor, Michigan
www.cherrylakepublishing.com

Content Adviser: Noshene Ranjbar, MD

Design: The Design Lab

Photo Credits: Cover and page 3, ©Marmaduke St. John/Alamy; page 4, ©Elliot Westacott, used
under license from Shutterstock, Inc.; page 6, ©Tetra Images/Alamy; page 9, ©sciencephotos/
Alamy; page 11, ©Oramstock/Alamy; page 13, ©Nucleus Medical Art, Inc./Alamy; page 14, ©The
Print Collector/Alamy; page 17, ©Steve Hamblin/Alamy; page 18, ©AP Photo/Gail Burton; page
19, ©Tom Tracy Photography/Alamy; page 22, ©AP Photo/The Missoulian, Tom Bauer; page
25, ©imagebroker/Alamy; page 26, ©Lebrecht Music and Arts Photo Library/Alamy; page 28,
©Edward Moss/Alamy; page 29, ©Medical-on-Line/Alamy

Library of Congress Cataloging-in-Publication Data
Gray, Susan Heinrichs.
 Hearing / by Susan H. Gray.
    p. cm.—(Innovation in medicine)
Includes index.
ISBN-13: 978-1-60279-227-2
ISBN-10: 1-60279-227-5
1. Hearing—Juvenile literature. I. Title. II. Series.
QP462.2.G74 2009
612.8'5—dc22   2008007716

Cherry Lake Publishing would like to acknowledge the work of
The Partnership for 21st Century Skills.
Please visit www.21stcenturyskills.org for more information.

CONTENTS

CHAPTER ONE

From Ear Trumpets to Transistors

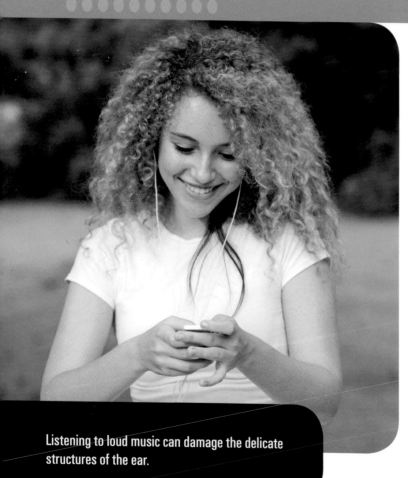

Listening to loud music can damage the delicate structures of the ear.

"Maria, what time do you have to be at basketball practice?" asked her mom.

"Maria? Maria?! Turn down that iPod!"

As her mother walked toward her, Maria looked up. "What?" she asked.

Her mom reached up and took one of the iPod earbuds out of Maria's ear. "You'd better turn the volume down on this thing. You haven't heard a word I said. You're going to damage your ears!"

Maria rolled her eyes. "Oh, Mom! You're just being dramatic."

"No, I'm not being dramatic. If you knew more about how your ears work, you might think twice about turning up the volume!"

A Greek doctor named Hippocrates (hih-PAHK-rah-tees) studied the eardrum 2,400 years ago. He was certain it was connected to hearing.

For about the next 2,000 years, scientists continued to learn about the ear. Still, they couldn't offer much help to anyone with hearing loss. In about 200 AD, another Greek doctor, Galen, wrote about nerves connecting the ears to the brain. In the 1500s, scientists described the tiny bones, muscles, canals, and other structures inside the ear.

Devices for those with hearing loss finally appeared in the 1600s. Ear trumpets and speaking tubes were the biggest innovations of the time. Ear trumpets were metal, horn-shaped devices. The user held the smaller end to the ear. The flared end was pointed toward a person speaking. Auricles were a pair of very small ear trumpets. They either looped over each ear or attached to a headband. People liked them because they were small and freed the user's hands.

Speaking tubes were much longer versions of ear trumpets. The speaker talked into a funnel at one end. The listener held the narrow end just inside his ear. Many variations existed. Some even had designs etched into the metal.

By 1700, doctors had a basic understanding of the ear's structure. They knew that sound enters the ear canal and makes the eardrum vibrate. They also knew that there were three tiny bones on the other side of the eardrum. They figured out that those bones picked up the vibrations. They also knew that the last bone carries vibrations to a hollow tube of the inner ear called the **cochlea**. Nerves run from the cochlea to the brain.

Still, there were many details to work out. The 19th century was a time of much learning and experimentation. By the end of the century, inventors in Germany had developed an instrument called an **otoscope**. Doctors could use this tool to look into ears.

The first electric hearing aids were introduced around 1900. Early models were large and expensive. They only helped those with mild hearing loss. But they paved the way for more advanced models.

In the 1920s, an American doctor named Harvey Fletcher developed an electrical device called the

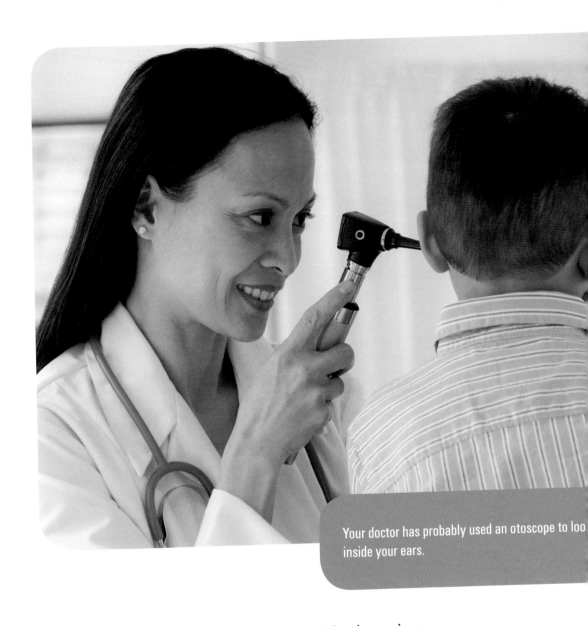

Your doctor has probably used an otoscope to loo[k] inside your ears.

audiometer. It measured hearing activity in patients. Now doctors could learn exactly how well patients could hear in each ear. They could also measure hearing loss over time.

About this same time, another invention came into use—the operating microscope. Doctors could look through its lenses and see the tiny structures of the ear greatly magnified. Using this instrument, they could perform delicate surgeries on the ear.

By 1945, scientists and doctors had made great strides in understanding the **anatomy** of the ear. It was good timing. Soldiers were returning from World War II (1939–1945). Many had some level of hearing loss. They had been exposed to loud explosions and gunfire with no ear protection during the war. So it was good that hearing aids were available. But most models were expensive. In addition, they required large batteries and vacuum tubes.

Vacuum tubes turn a weak electrical signal into a strong one. They were used to amplify sound. But the tubes were large and made of glass. They used a lot of energy, and heated up when in use. Vacuum-tube hearing aids caused many problems for those who used them.

Vacuum tubes were used in many other electrical devices, such as radios, television sets, and church organs. But they often burned out. So scientists looked for something more reliable to replace them. In 1947, a group of researchers invented the **transistor**. It amplified signals just as a vacuum tube did. But the transistor was smaller and sturdier than a vacuum tube. It also used less energy.

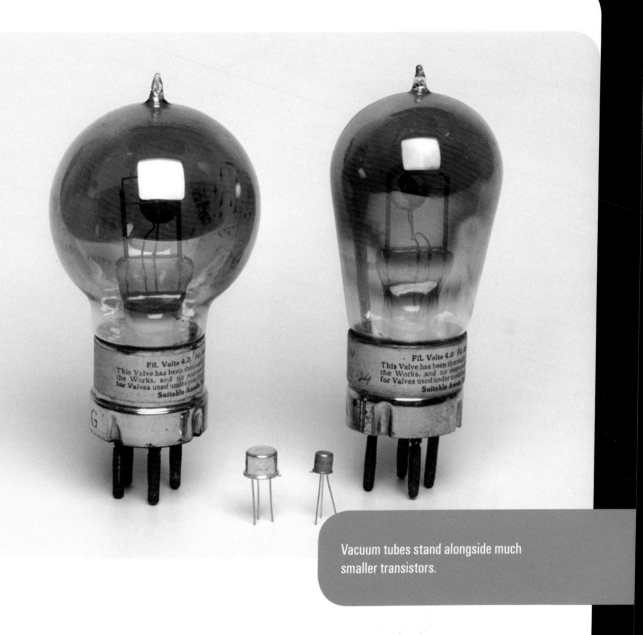

Vacuum tubes stand alongside much smaller transistors.

Soon most electronic devices used transistors. Hearing aids that were once barely able to fit into a pocket now fit right behind the ear.

Life & Career Skills

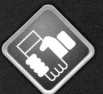

Many people know that Alexander Graham Bell invented the telephone. Few, however, know that he was also a champion of the deaf. Bell's lifelong interest in communication began at home. His mother had very poor hearing and used a speaking tube to hear people. Bell, however, spoke to her using a low voice, with his lips very close to her forehead. He believed his mother could hear him by sensing the vibrations in his voice.

As a young man, Bell got a job teaching deaf students to speak. He later fell in love with and married a student named Mabel Hubbard. Living with a deaf wife only strengthened his interest in communication.

In 1876, Bell and Thomas Watson succeeded in creating the first telephone. Bell gained much fame and fortune from this invention. But he always thought of himself as a teacher of the deaf. Successful innovators, such as Bell, use teamwork, creativity, and life experience to solve problems.

Audiometers, operating microscopes, and surgical procedures were constantly improving, too. Innovations in **otology** (the branch of medicine that deals with the ear) seemed to be coming faster and faster.

CHAPTER TWO

"A Boom Within the Head"

Some call it the "most exciting development in otology." They are speaking of the 20th-century innovation called cochlear implants. These devices allow some totally deaf people to hear sounds they couldn't hear before.

To understand how cochlear implants work, you need to understand how the ear works. Sound waves hitting the

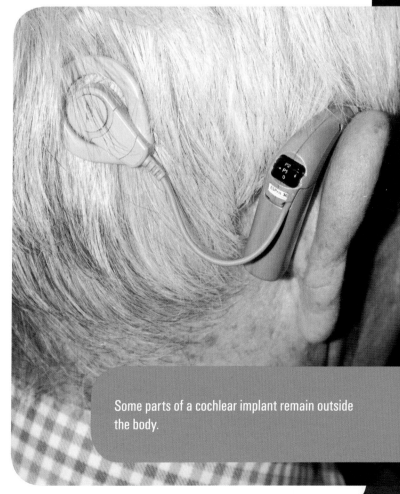

Some parts of a cochlear implant remain outside the body.

eardrum cause it to move back and forth, or vibrate. A tiny bone called the **malleus** is connected to the inside of the eardrum. The malleus rests against a bone called the **incus**. The incus rests against a third bone called the **stapes**. Beneath the stapes is a thin layer, or membrane, that covers a hole in the cochlea. When a sound enters the ear, it sets off a chain reaction. The eardrum, all three tiny bones, and the cochlear membrane begin to vibrate.

The cochlea is a hollow tube filled with fluid. It is coiled like a snail shell. Inside the cochlea are nerve cells that detect changes of pressure in the fluid. When the stapes vibrates against the cochlea, it causes changes in pressure. Nerve cells in the cochlea detect those changes and send electrical signals to the brain. The brain interprets the sound. All of these things happen in a fraction of a second.

Cochlear implants are devices that bypass the eardrum, the bones, and the hole in the cochlea. They pick up sound, turn it into electrical energy, and send electrical signals straight to the **auditory** nerve which carries them to the brain. Doctors started performing cochlear implant surgery in the 20th century. But the roots of this operation go back to the late 1700s and the work of Alessandro Volta.

Volta was an Italian scientist who worked with electricity. He is probably best known as the inventor of the battery. At one point, he wondered what would happen if he gave his own auditory system an electric jolt. Would it make him hear a sound? If so, what kind of sound?

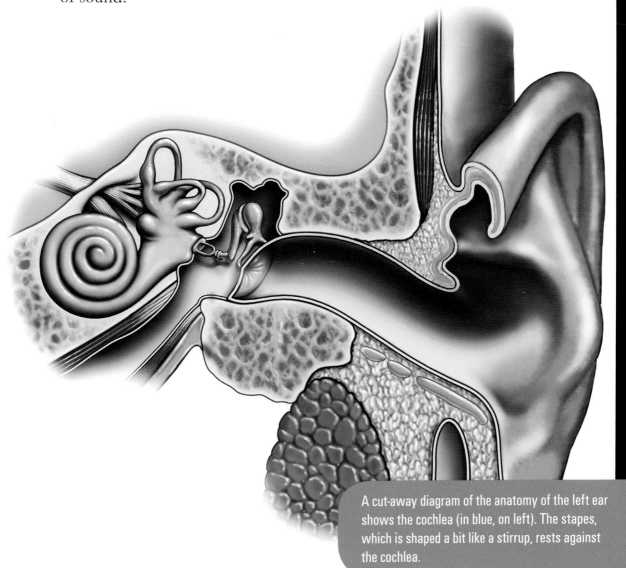

A cut-away diagram of the anatomy of the left ear shows the cochlea (in blue, on left). The stapes, which is shaped a bit like a stirrup, rests against the cochlea.

Volta connected two metal rods to a battery. Then he stuck the rods into his ears. Suddenly, he heard "a boom within the head." It was followed by a sound he described as the boiling of thick soup.

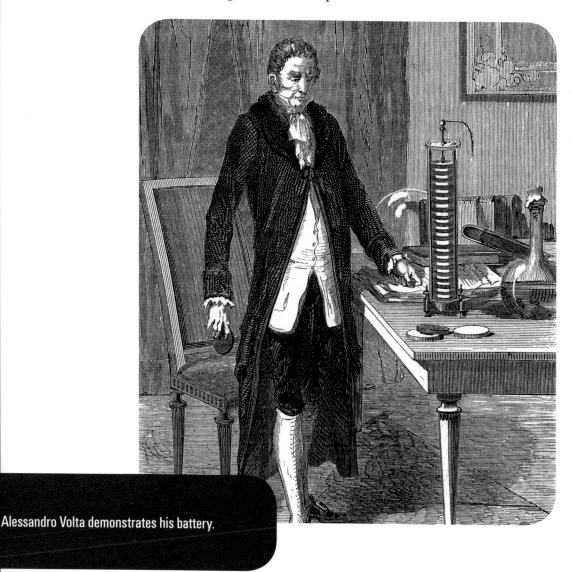

Alessandro Volta demonstrates his battery.

Volta was not the only one trying to create sound with electricity. Other scientists tried different versions of his experiment. They changed the strength of the electrical current. They also changed the placement of the metal rods. None of these experiments produced useful sounds. Most scientists eventually lost interest in trying.

Much later, though, interest returned. In 1957, two doctors operated on a completely deaf patient. They implanted a tiny device that could carry an electric current. The device touched a nerve in the patient's ear. After the surgery, the doctors set up a microphone and amplifier near the patient. The patient was able to make out sounds in his environment! The sounds, however, were not very clear.

Many scientists recognized the importance of this discovery. They began looking for ways to improve the device. They wanted to help the deaf hear. But hearing is a complex process. The ear picks up sounds and turns them into meaningful electrical impulses. Could they create a device to do all of that? They decided it was possible.

Some scientists developed a tiny microphone that could pick up sounds from a deaf patient's environment. They also created a speech processor to separate and arrange those sounds. They made the microphone and processor small enough to fit outside a deaf person's head.

Learning & Innovation Skills

Some people think that cochlear implants threaten the deaf way of life. They worry that the implants will cause deaf culture and sign language to disappear. These people have been deaf for much or all of their lives. They communicate with sign language. But they also live, go to school, and work with people who hear. They don't consider themselves disabled in any way. They don't want people to think that deaf people need to be "fixed."

Many other people disagree. They believe that no one should be denied the opportunity to improve his or her hearing. They believe that children who receive the implants will do better in life. What do you think?

In the meantime, other scientists built a receiver. It picked up signals from the speech processor and turned them into electrical impulses. They also developed a packet of wires to carry the electrical signals to the auditory nerve. The receiver and wires were small enough to be surgically placed inside a patient's head.

This four-part device— microphone, speech processor, receiver, and wires—is now called a cochlear implant. It was first tried on deaf patients in the 1970s. Scientists have improved it many times since then. Patients with the device don't hear perfectly. They often still rely on sign language and speech reading. But they hear well enough to get along in the hearing world. Today, thousands of people around the world are living with cochlear implants.

CHAPTER THREE

More Innovations

Cochlear implants have produced amazing results. But they are not the only hearing innovation in use today. Doctors have also learned how to replace damaged ear bones, for example. And engineers have created some remarkable hearing aids.

Sometimes people lose their hearing because the stapes does not work properly. When too much bone tissue grows in the

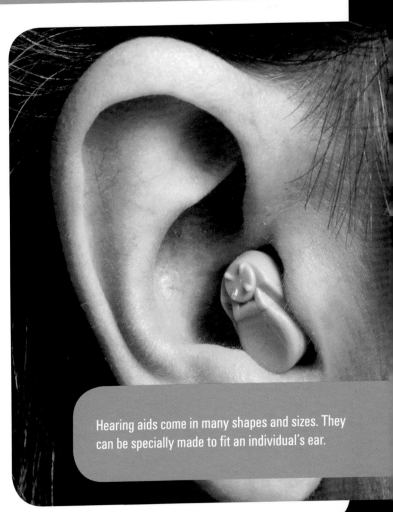

Hearing aids come in many shapes and sizes. They can be specially made to fit an individual's ear.

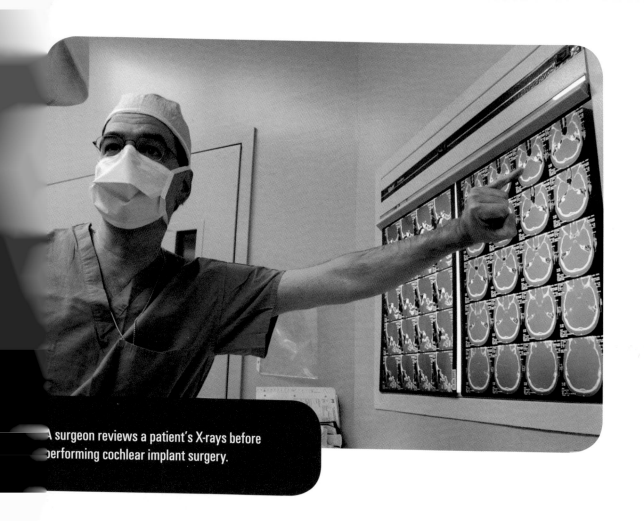

A surgeon reviews a patient's X-rays before performing cochlear implant surgery.

middle ear, the stapes locks up. Then it doesn't vibrate against the cochlea. People with this problem slowly become deaf.

Before the 1900s, doctors did not know exactly what caused this kind of deafness. They sometimes tried to cure it by removing the eardrum, malleus, incus, and stapes. In time, they stopped doing this surgery. They decided that it did more harm than good.

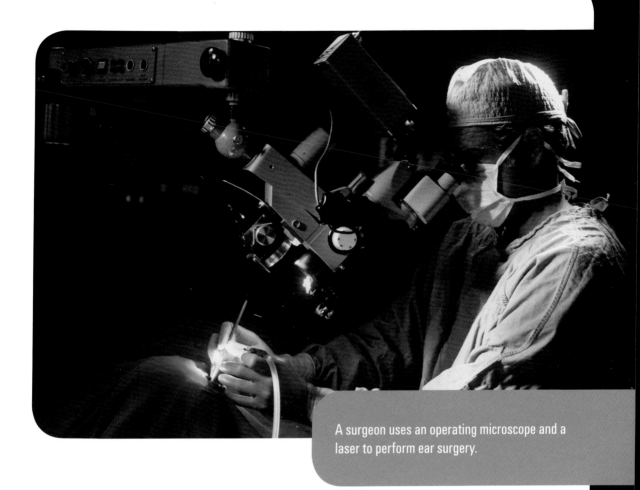

A surgeon uses an operating microscope and a laser to perform ear surgery.

The operating microscope was invented in the 20th century. Better audiometers were also designed. These tools helped doctors learn more about the stapes and how it works. One doctor found that loosening the stapes improved his patient's hearing immediately. Another found that replacing the stapes with an artificial one also worked. Today, stapes replacement restores hearing to many people each year.

21st Century Content

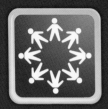 One-year-old Helen Keller got very sick in 1882. The illness left her both deaf and blind. But that didn't stop her. Over the next 25 years, she learned sign language, studied, and graduated from college with the highest honors. Then she devoted her life to helping blind and deaf-blind people. She became famous for her remarkable achievements. She died in 1968, but her life continues to inspire people around the world.

Today, the Helen Keller Institute for the Deaf and Deafblind in India educates children with severe hearing and vision issues. New York City's Helen Keller International works to prevent blindness and poor nutrition worldwide. These organizations make a difference in the lives of many people in need. "Although the world is full of suffering," Helen Keller once said, "it is also full of the overcoming of it."

Some people with poor hearing need only a hearing aid. Transistors helped shrink the size of hearing aids. But many people were still unhappy with them. They said the aids picked up too many loud sounds. They also complained that the hearing aids were uncomfortable to wear. Engineers listened to their complaints and worked to find solutions. Eventually, they came up with tiny hearing aids that amplify soft sounds but not loud ones. They also developed molded hearing aids to fit each patient's ear canal. Researchers continue to look for ways to improve hearing aid design and technology.

CHAPTER FOUR

The Future of Otology

Scientists in the field of otology have great hopes for the future. Some are looking for ways to regrow damaged nerves. They are studying the use of chemicals produced by some of the body's glands. These chemicals are called growth **hormones**. They hope that the chemicals will help repair auditory nerves that are injured in accidents or damaged by disease.

Other doctors and engineers are researching ways to improve cochlear implants. They are trying to develop implants that give clearer, sharper hearing. They also want to make the implants smaller. They are also working to find ways to make cochlear implant surgery more affordable. Today, cochlear implants are too expensive for many people.

Research areas in otology are varied. Some scientists are working to understand hearing loss that runs in

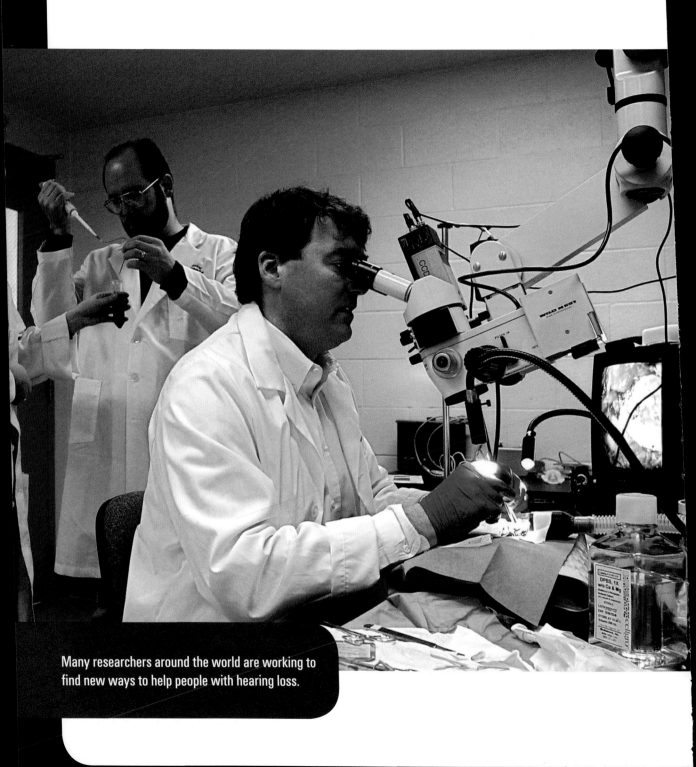

Many researchers around the world are working to find new ways to help people with hearing loss.

families. Others are trying to create better and more lifelike artificial ear bones. Engineers are working on hearing aids that can recognize the difference between a human voice and other sounds. All of their work promises a future filled with innovation in the field of otology.

Learning & Innovation Skills

Gallaudet University is a school for deaf students in Washington, D.C. Some people say that its football players invented the huddle in 1894. They realized that the other team could read their sign language when they gathered to discuss their next play. To keep their plans a secret, the players began to form huddles. The practice quickly caught on with other teams, the story goes, and before long, the huddle became a part of every football game. What else has the deaf community given the hearing world?

CHAPTER FIVE

A Few Giants in the Field

Every modern-day innovation in medicine builds on the work of earlier researchers. This is certainly true in otology. For example, no one could have developed a cochlear implant before someone else identified the cochlea and how it works.

Bartolomeo Eustachius

Bartolomeo Eustachius was an early researcher of human anatomy. He lived in Italy in the 1500s. At the time, scientists were just beginning to understand human anatomy. They closely examined human bodies, including organs and tissues, and made very detailed drawings.

Eustachius wrote a book on human anatomy, including a special section on the ear. He explained that the malleus, incus, and stapes were related to hearing.

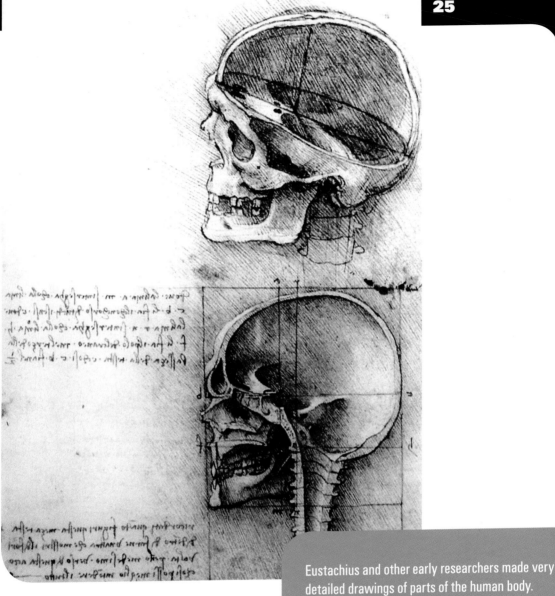

Eustachius and other early researchers made very detailed drawings of parts of the human body.

He also described the tube that runs from the middle ear down to the throat. That tube is now known as the Eustachian tube. Eustachius laid the groundwork for the doctors who came after him.

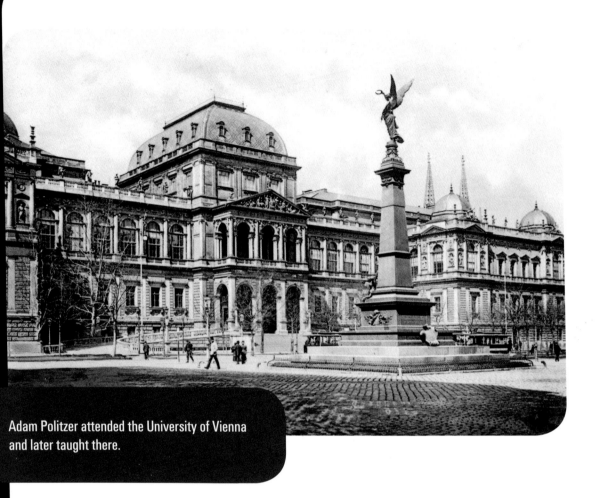

Adam Politzer attended the University of Vienna and later taught there.

Adam Politzer

Born in Hungary in 1835, Adam Politzer always had a hunger for learning. As a young doctor, he became interested in the ear and related diseases. He was also a skilled artist and spoke several languages. During his life, he cared for patients and taught medical students. He also developed instruments for examining and treating the ear and wrote books on ear diseases.

As his fame spread, patients from distant countries came to him for treatment. Fortunately, he was able to communicate in their languages. He also worked in his town's poorhouses and nursing homes. This helped him learn even more about ear diseases and the best treatments for them. Politzer was constantly learning and passing his knowledge on to others. Today, people consider his books among the great works in otology.

Graeme Clark

Dr. Graeme Clark of Australia is a modern-day innovator who has helped thousands of people to hear. He was always interested in science and enjoyed reading about the achievements of innovative people.

As a boy, Clark worked in his deaf father's drugstore. Later, as a medical student, he realized that he wanted to help deaf people. He wondered if an electronic ear could help them hear. He began work on this idea in 1967.

Life & Career Skills

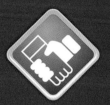

Ear surgeons were some of the first doctors to use the operating microscope. Doctors use this microscope when they are operating on extremely small parts of the body. Without operating microscopes, surgeons run a greater risk of damaging a patient's hearing.

Today, surgeons in many different fields use the operating microscope. It is used for reattaching arms, legs, or fingers severed in accidents. It is also used for eye surgery and for removing tumors from the brain and spinal cord. Many innovations come from adapting tools, such as the operating microscope, for new uses.

Other doctors thought his dream was hopeless, but that didn't stop him. He even quit his job as a doctor to work on the electronic ear.

Clark worked on his project for years. Sometimes he had barely enough money to keep going. He was often criticized by other doctors. But he continued his work.

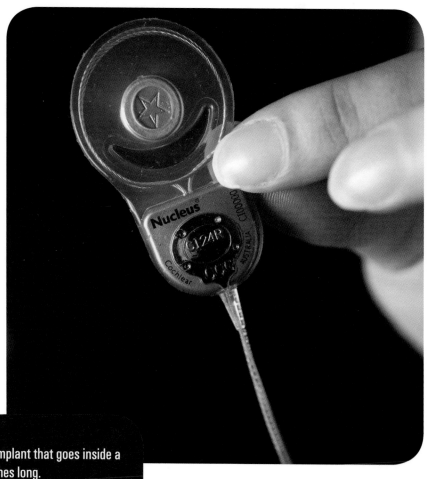

The portion of a cochlear implant that goes inside a patient's head is a few inches long.

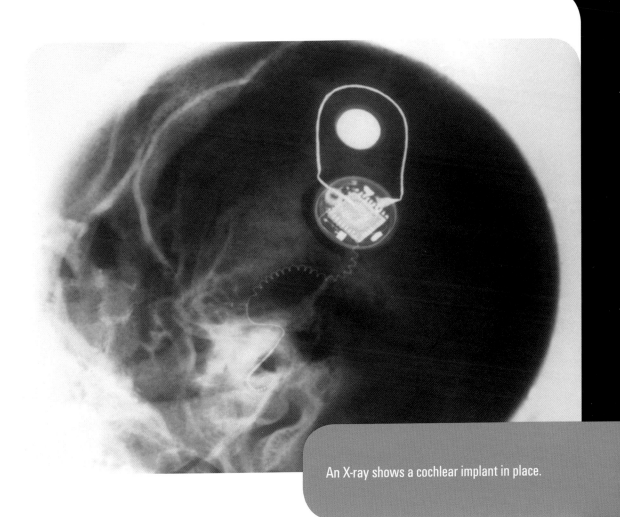

An X-ray shows a cochlear implant in place.

Finally, in 1978, Clark implanted his electronic ear in a patient. When the man was able to hear after the surgery, Clark went into another room and cried with joy.

It took years of commitment, creative thinking, and hard work, but his efforts paid off. Clark's cochlear implant has helped deaf children and adults all over the world.

Glossary

anatomy (uh-NAT-uh-mee) the structure of living things

audiometer (aw-dee-OHM-et-ur) an electrical device that measures hearing activity

auditory (AW-dih-tor-ee) having to do with hearing

cochlea (KOKE-lee-uh) a hollow tube of the inner ear with the nerve endings necessary to hear; it is usually coiled like a snail shell

hormones (HORE-monz) chemicals produced by some of the body's glands that affect growth and development

incus (EENG-kuss) one of three small bones in the ear between the malleus and the stapes

malleus (MAL-ee-uss) the outermost bone of three small bones in the ear

middle ear (MID-uhl IR) the part of the ear that houses the malleus, incus, and stapes

otology (oh-TAL-uh-jee) the branch of medicine that deals with the ear

otoscope (OH-tuh-skope) an instrument for looking at the inside of the ear

stapes (STAY-peez) the innermost bone of three small bones in the ear

transistor (tran-ZISS-tur) a small electronic device that controls the flow of electricity in equipment such as radios and television sets

For More Information

BOOKS

Carson, Mary Kay. *Alexander Graham Bell: Giving Voice to the World*. New York: Sterling, 2007.

Libal, Autumn. *The Ocean Inside: Youth Who Are Deaf and Hard of Hearing*. Broomall, PA: Mason Crest Publishers, 2004.

Sullivan, George. *Helen Keller: Her Life in Pictures*. New York: Scholastic Nonfiction, 2006.

Zoll, Andrea J., and Arlene J. Garcia. *Luke and His Hearing-Ear Dog, Herald*. Victoria, B.C.: Trafford Publishing, 2006.

WEB SITES

ASL for Kids
library.thinkquest.org/5875/
Information about American Sign Language

Helen Keller Kids Museum Online
www.afb.org/braillebug/helen_keller_bio.asp
For a kids' page about Helen Keller

Neuroscience for Kids
faculty.washington.edu/chudler/bigear.html
To find out more about ear anatomy and how the ear works

Index

About the Author

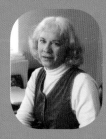

Susan H. Gray has a master's degree in zoology. She has taught college-level courses in biology, anatomy, and physiology. She also has written more than 90 science and reference books for children. In her free time, she likes to garden and play the piano. Susan lives in Cabot, Arkansas, with her husband, Michael, and many pets.